THE ERECTILE
DYSFUNCTION
FIX

HOW TO REGAIN SEXUAL FUNCTION, LIBIDO AND TREAT ERECTILE DYSFUNCTION WITHOUT DRUGS OR SURGERY WITH PLATELET RICH PLASMA, THE PRIAPUS SHOT® (P-SHOT®)

Anne Truong, MD

10340 Spotsylvania Avenue, Suite 101
Fredericksburg, VA 22408
(540) 374-3164

www.Truongrehab.com
Facebook: truongrehabilitationcenter
Twitter: @truongrehab

ISBN 13: 978-19-805-4894-2

TABLE OF CONTENTS

If you want to learn more about Platelets Rich Plasma and its healing power go to:

https://bit.ly/regenyou

To learn more about how to live pain-free, look and feel younger, regain your libido, enjoy sex, and work more efficiently, go to:

https://bit.ly/rejuvyou

DISCLAIMER

This material has been written and published solely for educational purposes. The publisher and author make no representation or warranties with respect to accuracy or completeness of the content of this work and specifically disclaim all warranties. The author and the publisher will neither have liability or responsibility to any person with respect to any loss, damage, or injury caused or alleged to be caused directly or indirectly by the information in this book. The intent of this book is not to dispense medical advice or prescribe the use of any techniques as a formal treatment for any physical medical conditions or psychological or emotional problems, without advice of a physician either directly or indirectly taking care of the individual. The intent of this book is to offer information and to help the reader be more informed to make wise choices for their medical care. The author assumes no responsibility if you choose to use any of the information in this book. Statements made in this book have not been evaluated by the Food and Drug Administration. The content of this book is not intended to diagnose or treat any condition, illness, or disease. Individual experience will be unique with variable results.

DEDICATION

The book is dedicated to my husband, Bao, and my two children, Ryan and Kelsey. Without their support, I would not be where I am today. I thank you for your unconditional love.

ACKNOWLEDGMENT

I would like to thank Dr. Charles Runels, developer of the Priapus Shot®, called the P Shot®, and the Orgasm Shot® called the O Shot®. Additionally, he created the Vampire Facial®, Vampire Facelift®, Vampire Breast Lift®, and Vampire Hair Regrowth® trademarked procedures. His innovation and creativity have improved many patients' quality of life and have given physicians the opportunity to change lives as they have never done before. His generosity and mentorship inspired me to write this book, and I am grateful for Dr. Runels' support.

INTRODUCTION

I am living the American dream. I came to the United States as a Vietnamese refugee in 1975 during the Vietnam War. My family was prosperous and affluent in Saigon. We had a vacation home, and I went to private schools driven by chauffeurs. When my family of eight emigrated to the US, we had nothing but the clothes on our backs. We were lucky, and we're gratified that we are together and have new lives. My father had a college degree at the University of Michigan, spoke five languages, and was once an affluent politician, had to work as a grocery clerk to feed his family. My mom, who never worked in her entire life worked in housekeeping at a local hotel. Those of my siblings who were over 16 years old had to work after school. All our incomes were put into one bank account to support the whole family. The children didn't have much, but we didn't mind, as we learned that one had to earn what they had in life. You don't take anything for granted. I took the bus everywhere and worked in high school. I took out loans and worked in college after classes. I wanted to be a doctor because I love to help people and make a difference. My grandfather was a doctor in Vietnam. School, work, and life in general were not easy, but it made me into a stronger person. I took out loans for medical school and I knew it was my calling.

Living on borrowed money, I had to budget carefully, as it was not enough for food, lodging, and books. Eating out was a luxury I couldn't afford. A box of ramen noodles was often my daily nutrition as it was cheap and lasted weeks. When my husband and I got married at the end of medical school, everything we owned could fit into our 1986 two car door Nissan Sentra. These struggling times created a lot of great memories. It made me more determined to reach my goal of the being a Physiatrist.

A Physiatrist is a medical doctor specializing in Physical Medicine and Rehabilitation. This specialty requires one year of training in Internal Medicine or Surgery and three years training in a Physical Medicine and Rehabilitation residency program. A Physiatrist treats a wide variety of medical conditions affecting the brain, spinal cord, nerves, bones, joints, ligaments, muscles, and tendons.

I earned my Biology degree from University of California at Berkeley and then worked as a medical researcher at the University of California at San Francisco in the liver transplant department. This work ignited my interests in stem cell therapy and cellular regeneration. I attended medical school at The University of Nevada in Reno and Las Vegas, and I completed my Physical Medicine and Rehabilitation residency program at Baylor College of Medicine in Houston, Texas.

I feel that treating a condition must be more than just giving medication or recommending surgery. I want to make an impact by treating the source of the problem. I want to develop a better protocol that can reverse and heal the body and not just address the symptoms of the problem.

I treat the patient's pain without opioids, pain medication, and surgery. I evaluate the patient as a whole person and try to address pain with rehabilitation and nonsurgical treatment techniques first, with the goal of improving quality of life. I treat the source of the problem and not the symptoms of prolonged and reversible diseases. I stress education, rehabilitation, and regenerative therapies to achieve this outcome without using medications and avoiding surgeries.

Medication addresses the symptoms; it is synthetic, but it does not heal the condition. For instance, if you have high blood pressure, you take medication to control your blood pressure. The medication does not cure you of having high blood pressure; it just lowers it, thus preventing the symptoms and consequences of high blood pressure. Without the medication, you continue to have high blood pressure. For instance, weight loss can cure nonfamilial high blood pressure. A family history of a disease puts you at risk, but your body and your lifestyle can modify the outcome of the risk factor.

Over the course of my career, I became a functional medicine and a regenerative medicine practitioner. In 2007, I started doing platelet-rich plasma (PRP) for musculoskeletal conditions (e.g. arthritis pain in joints, injured tendons and ligaments) and subsequently added regenerative cell therapies such as bone marrow and fat cell therapy in addition to PRP. I then transitioned to using PRP for aesthetic and sexual dysfunctions. The transition is the best decision I ever made, and I have to thank Dr. Charles Runels and Dr. Kathleen Posey for making this happen.

As a regenerative medicine and a functional medicine practitioner, when you regenerate and rejuvenate tissues, you are also improving the release of hormones, neurotransmitters, and causing important cellular processes. The impaired tissue is surrounded with healing factors to promote cellular healing in order to restore tissue to its natural function. This method is the most effective treatment for the source of the problem, from musculoskeletal injuries and injuries to soft tissues such as muscles and ligaments, to rejuvenating the face and fixing sexual dysfunction.

One of the most gratifying conditions to treat is sexual dysfunction. This has not been at the forefront of research and novel treatment. Often, sexuality is neglected during the doctor's visit. The Priapus Shot ® is using Platelet Rich Plasma (PRP) to treat male erectile dysfunction and Peyronie's disease. The Orgasm Shot ® (O Shot®) is using PRP for female urinary stress incontinence and sexual dysfunction. Treating these conditions will not only improve the patient's sexual functions, but it also can improve and/or repair the patient's relationship and life. This book is intended to provide men and their partners a resource for erectile dysfunction. Erectile dysfunction can be treated with the least invasive method, the Priapus Shot ®. This book can be used by the providers of the Priapus Shot®as a resource for their patients with erectile dysfunction. The goal is to dispense information to the patient and to the providers to try the Priapus Shot® as an alternative or as a complement to medication.

FOREWORD

You and I both needed Dr. Anne Truong to write this book. I'll explain.

Eighteen years ago, while serving as the medical director of a hospital-based wound care center, I began thinking about ideas that would eventually lead to the injection of my own penis with PRP and to my eventual design of the Priapus Shot® procedure. I did this, initially, in secret because I feared the repercussion of attempting to bring such an idea to the medical establishment.

When I saw the benefits of the procedure for me and for my patients, I started looking for physician teachers & researchers who would act with intelligence, good judgment, and bravery—perhaps most importantly, bravery, since any new idea will meet attack by the brain with the same force that a foreign protein will meet attack by the immune system.

So, when I met Dr. Truong and she used her experience to think deeply about the Priapus Shot® procedure and then when she offered to teach others the nuances of the technique, I was very grateful. Dr. Truong's expertise in tissue repair and rehabilitation make her uniquely stellar in her ability to move the ideas of the Priapus Shot® procedure forward. And, it's the movement of ideas forward that make them most useful.

Dr. Truong—having served as a professor at her local Medical College and having published research in the areas of tissue repair—brings unique skills and attitudes to our mission of teaching the world a better way to vitalize or to rehabilitate the penis.

Though emotionally the genitals bring thoughts of sacred protection and ideas of untouchable territory, the blood vessels and the nerves and collagen of the penis grow and heal in the same way as do the nerve and blood vessels and collagen of other parts of the body. Dr. Truong's experience and research in rehabilitating people from the worst of injuries bring a very helpful perspective.

So, I am immensely grateful for Dr. Truong's thoughtfulness and courage to bring to you this treatise on ways you might improve penile health and function.

I encourage you to read thoughtfully and to contact Dr Truong. Physicians will grow under her instruction. Men will heal under her care. And, since sex brings much more than pleasure, since sex affects creativity, intelligence, and family relations, because of this book, lives will profoundly change.

I hope that one of those lives will be yours.

Charles Runels, MD
Inventor of the Priapus Shot® procedure

Chapter 1:

MYTHS, AND TESTIMONIALS OF THE PRIAPUS SHOT®

MYTHS

There are a lot of misconceptions about erectile dysfunction. Being well-informed is the best way to avoid taking supplements or "pills" that may not help your ED but may harm you.

Some common myths are:

1. Younger men can have ED, but not as frequently as older men do.

    A Study in The American Journal of Medicine (69) found in men ages 20-39, 15% have at least occasional difficulty with erections during sex. In the 40-59 age group, 12 % sometimes have difficulty with erections, and 2% cannot have an erection at all.

2. If you can have an erection, you don't have erectile dysfunction.

    Erectile Dysfunction (ED) is the inability for a man to maintain an erection for satisfying sexual relations. Symptoms can also include struggling to maintain an erection for long enough to complete intercourse or an inability to ejaculate. A man can get an erection but may not have been able to maintain penetration.

3. Erectile dysfunction is all mental.

    Erectile dysfunction is physical, mental and environmental. Problems with high blood pressure, diabetes, blood flow dysfunction, weight gain, hormonal imbalance, and smoking can affect blood flow to the penis. Often, ED is an indication of existing circulation problems before it becomes symptomatic. ED is a warning to see the doctor for an evaluation before you start taking "enhancements" on your own. Getting a consultation with a doctor may save your life.

    Your lifestyle may impact on erection capacity. Smoking, illicit drugs, obesity, alcohol can adversely affect erections.

    Often, treating ED encompasses correcting lifestyle choices, optimizing hormones, the use of a pump, and, if needed, a reduced dose of medication.

4S. Medications are the only treatment; if you don't respond to this, you are out of luck.

There are multiple options available. Testosterone replacement is given as an intramuscular injection, in topical form, as well as in patches, troches (small, medicated lozenges) and in pellets. There is intra-penile injection with alprostadil, or Trimix. A penis pump is another option. And lastly, penis implants. The Priapus Shot® is the best option. This book will discuss these options further. These may be less costly than medications like Viagra.

TESTIMONIALS

PATIENT #1

Patient #1 is 53 years old and is a recently divorced man who has Peyronie's Disease. The bend in his penis was not painful, but he was unable to get fully erect compared to when he was younger. His libido was declining as well his sense of well-being. He felt he was not "performing" as well as he could. He felt insecure with women and often avoided dating. He felt hopeless and wanted a new life and outlook.

He hoped the Priapus Shot® would decrease the bending, thicken his shaft, and increase his libido. He received the Priapus Shot® about four years ago (also taking testosterone) and it indeed decreased the bending of the penis and thickened his shaft. The P Shot® increased his confidence and his libido to pursue a new relationship. He is still in a long-term relationship. He feels the P Shot® improved his quality of life and is completely satisfied with the outcome. Patient #1 recommends the P Shot® to anyone who wants to improve his sex life.

Patient #2

Patient #2 is 47 years old and has been married for 23 years. His marriage is not the same as it used to be; he doesn't bond with the wife as much, and they don't spend a lot of time together. As a result, Patient #2 is temporarily separated. He was taking anti-depression medications and started drinking heavily. He gained weight. This spiraling lifestyle exacerbated his libido and erection. He wanted to do something but didn't know where to start. He wanted to do the Priapus Shot® to see if it could improve his libido and erectile dysfunction. Three months later, he stopped all medications, quit drinking and moved back with his wife, and they are happier than ever. He said the Priapus Shot® saved his life and marriage.

Patient #3

Patient #3 is a 68-year-old man who has been married for 45 years. He had a history of erectile dysfunction for at least ten years. He had been taking Viagra, at first at a 25mg dose, but had since increased to 50mg. He can get firmness about a quarter of the time; the rest of the time he does not get firmness. The medication does not last as long as it used to. He does not like the loss of spontaneity and planning of his sex life. He has to fast for 1-2 hours and take the medication 1-2 hours before intercourse. He is happily married and wanted to please his wife emotionally and physically.

He loves his wife. He wanted to show her he still desires her. They don't have intimacy anymore because of his erectile dysfunction. Both he and his wife are on hormonal replacement therapies and are both physically active. He wanted to do the Priapus Shot® for erectile dysfunction. After receiving the Priapus Shot® and using the vacuum pump, within three weeks, he was able to get a full erection every time with half a 25mg Viagra pill. By three months, he was thrilled to feel "vitality" again. He and his wife now have a great relationship like they had when they first married.

Chapter 2:

IT'S NOT JUST ABOUT SEX

Arelationship is an emotional and a physical component that bonds two people together. Love is defined by Merriam Webster as a feeling of a deep romantic or sexual attachment to someone. Sexual intimacy is the key to a pleasurable and emotional bond with your partner. Unfortunately, as we age, sexual functions and libido decline. Often, we think it is inevitable, irreversible, and part of aging. That is not the truth at all! There are treatments to improve sexual intimacy and slow down the aging process. You can feel like you are in your thirties again.

The decline in sexual response in a relationship can change the relationship as a whole. This change in intimacy can lead to the negative interpretation that the relationship is lacking.

Sexual pleasure is integral in a relationship. Any therapy or idea that enhances the sensation of any part of the body could contribute to an enhanced orgasm response during intimacy. Sexual intimacy enhances the relationship.

When a couple first meets, a physical attraction starts and then the emotional bond develops. This is what bonds them together initially and is an integral part of their love. Sexual intimacy is essential to bond and grow with our partner.

Treating erectile dysfunction not only improves a man's sexual function and increases libido, but it repairs and improves relationship issues. The treatment can return a couple to the beginning of their relationship and reignite their love for one another. Treating erectile dysfunction is more than just about sex; it is about love and relationship.

The Priapus Shot ® is a nonsurgical approach that can restore libido and erectile function for a man. This book will help you understand erectile dysfunction, treatment options, and discover the greatness of autologous Platelet Rich Plasma in your blood. The Priapus Shot® will change your life.

Chapter 3:

WHAT IS ERECTILE DYSFUNCTION?

What is An Erection?

The sympathetic nervous system maintains the flaccid penis. An erection starts when the brain sends neurotransmitter chemical messages to the arteries of the penis to increase blood flow. The arteries open up more extensively, which then allows the spongy tissue at the penis to be engorged; this engorgement of the tissue compresses the veins that lie between the two fascia layers of the penis. This mechanism compresses outflow of blood from the veins; the blood is then trapped in the spongy tissue of the penis called the corpus cavernosum. The blood outflow expands the penis and creates an erection. When the blood drains out to the veins, the penis becomes flaccid again.

WHAT IS ERECTILE DYSFUNCTION?

Erectile Dysfunction (ED) is the inability for a man to maintain an erection for satisfying sexual relations. Symptoms can also include struggling to maintain an erection for long enough to complete intercourse or an inability to ejaculate.

A man is considered to have ED when these symptoms occur regularly.

The normal male sexual function requires interactions among vascular, neurologic, hormonal, and psychological systems. The initial obligatory event required for male sexual activity, the acquisition and maintenance of penile erection, is primarily a vascular phenomenon, triggered by neurologic signals and facilitated only in the presence of an appropriate hormonal milieu and psychological mindset.

Psychogenic erection is triggered by nerves in the brain to the spinal cord to the blood vessels in the pelvis to the penis.

Touch stimulus creates reflex erections to the penis or genital area which initiates a reflex within the sacral nerve roots (sacrum 2-4, the sacral erection center).

Nocturnal erections occur only during rapid eye movement (REM) sleep [5]. Men who sleep fitfully and depressed men rarely experience REM sleep and do not have nocturnal or early morning erections.

Psychogenic erections are more common during man's early sexually active years, and a reflex erection occurs in the mature years.

The absolute prerequisites for penile erectile activity are an adequate arterial inflow to provide a constant source of intracavernosal (intra–penile muscle) oxygen and sufficient nitric oxide synthase to generate nitric oxide. Nitric oxide acts by promoting the generation of cyclic guanosine monophosphate (GMP). Detumescence (loss of erection) occurs when nitric oxide-induced vasodilation disappears because of metabolism of cyclic GMP, which is mediated by intracavernosal type 5 cyclic GMP phosphodiesterase [4]. Detumescence also is regulated in part by norepinephrine pathways.

The role of nitric oxide may have significant therapeutic implications for patients with Erectile Dysfunction (ED). Low intra-penile tissue nitric oxide synthase levels are found in cigarette smokers and patients with diabetes and testosterone deficiency, which may explain why these factors are associated with a high frequency of ED. On the other hand, sildenafil, as well as vardenafil, tadalafil, and avanafil, are all phosphodiesterase (PDE-5) inhibitors and help with increased flow. All four PDE-5 inhibitors enhance intracavernosal cyclic GMP levels to improve the erectile response to sexual stimulation in many men with ED.

Interference with oxygen delivery or nitric oxide synthesis can prevent intracavernosal blood pressure from rising to a level sufficient to impede venous outflow, leading to an inability to acquire or sustain a rigid erection. Examples include decreased blood flow and inadequate intracavernosal oxygen levels when atherosclerosis involves the hypogastric artery or other feeder vessels [5].

Chapter 4:

INCIDENCE AND PREVALENCE OF ERECTILE DYSFUNCTION (ED)

Erectile Dysfunction (ED) affects as many as 30 million men in the United States. Several studies have looked at the prevalence of ED. The Massachusetts Male Aging Study [1] reported ED in 52% of patients. The study demonstrated that ED is increasingly prevalent with age. At age 40, approximately 40% of men are affected. The rate increases to nearly 70% in men age 70 years. The prevalence of complete ED increases from 5% to 15% as age increases from 40 to 70 years. From this study, there would be approximately 30 million men in the United States with some form of erectile impairment. Age was the number one risk factor.

It means that there are about 617,715 new ED cases a year in the United States. If you have diabetes or hypertension, your risk is 57% for ED.

Following adjustment for age, a higher probability was in patients with heart disease, hypertension, diabetes, and those taking associated medications. Cigarette smoking in this study did not correlate with a higher likelihood of complete ED. However, when it was with heart disease and hypertension, a higher probability of ED was noted.

A larger national study, the National Health and Social Life Survey [2], looked at sexual function in men and women. Men in poor physical and emotional health experience more sexual dysfunction. It was concluded that sexual dysfunction is an important public health concern and added that emotional issues are likely to contribute to the experience of these problems.

Chapter 5:

RISK FACTORS FOR ERECTILE DYSFUNCTION (ED)

The normal male sexual function requires interactions among four systems: the neurologic, hormonal, psychological, and vascular. Erection is triggered by nerves in the brain which are relayed to the thoracolumbar erection center (thoracic spine level 11 to lumbar level 2). This impulse is directed to the vascular bed in the pelvis then into the corpora cavernosa (penis shaft tissue).

The four systems must work in harmony to achieve a full erection. Any disruption or imbalance in these systems will cause erectile dysfunction.

Men and women in good health are more sexually active compared to those in poor health. Interestingly, men lost more years of sexual activity due to poor health compared to women.

Men who present these risk factors are questioned about the presence of Erectile Dysfunction (ED).

Etiologies of Erectile Dysfunction[3]:

- Vascular:
  - ❖ Cardiovascular disease, atherosclerosis causes a narrowing or clogging of arteries in the penis, preventing the necessary blood flow to the penis to produce an erection.
  - ❖ Hypertension, diabetes mellitus, hyperlipidemia, smoking, major surgery (radical prostatectomy) or radiotherapy (pelvis or retroperitoneum)
- Neurologic: Spinal cord and brain injuries, Parkinson disease, Alzheimer's disease, multiple sclerosis, stroke
- Local penile (cavernous) factors: Peyronie's disease, cavernous fibrosis, penile fracture
- Hormonal: Hypogonadism, hyperprolactinemia, hyper- and hypothyroidism, hyper- and hypocortisolism, diabetes mellitus, adrenal disorders, chronic liver disease, chronic renal failure, and AIDS.
- Drug-induced: Antihypertensives, antidepressants, antipsychotics, antiandrogens, recreational drugs, opioid pain medications
- Psychogenic: Performance-related anxiety, past traumatic experiences, relationship problems, anxiety, depression, stress

- Lifestyle: Obesity, smoking, watching television, obstructive sleep apnea, restless leg syndrome
- Other: Systemic sclerosis (scleroderma), Peyronie's disease, and prostate cancer treatment (e.g., brachytherapy, prostatectomy).

ED usually develops from a mix of psychogenic and organic factors [4]:

- If a person is unable to get an erection with a sexual partner, but can achieve an erection during masturbation, or may find that they wake up with an erection, the cause of their impotence is most likely psychological.
- If a person is never able to get an erection, the cause of their impotence is most likely physical.

The lowest prevalence of ED was noted in men without chronic medical problems who engaged in healthy behaviors. In obese men with ED, weight loss and increased physical activity are associated with an improvement in erectile function in about one-third of patients [3].

The frequency of sexual activity appears to predict the development of ED. After adjusting for the simultaneous presence of chronic diseases in a patient (comorbidities) and other major risk factors, men who reported intercourse less than once per week developed ED at twice the rate as men who reported intercourse once per week [4].

Physical causes account for 90% of ED cases, with psychological causes much less common.

Psychological causes (4):

- In rare cases, a man may always have had ED and may never have achieved an erection. The condition is called Primary Erectile Dysfunction, and the cause is almost always psychological if there is no obvious anatomical deformity or physiological issue.
- guilt
- fear of intimacy
- depression
- severe anxiety

Most cases of ED are secondary. It means that erectile function has been normal, but becomes problematic. Causes of a new and persistent problem are usually physical.

There is overlap between medical and psychosocial causes. If a man is obese, blood flow changes can affect his ability to maintain an erection, which is a physical cause. However, he may also have low self-esteem, which can impact erectile function and is a psychosocial cause.

The most recent study[10] to investigate this found that there was no link between riding a bike and ED, but it did find an association between longer hours of cycling and the risk of prostate cancer.

Prostate cancer does not cause ED, but the surgery does.

Although sexual dysfunction is more common in older men, it also affects younger men (ages 18 to 25 years)[4].

Chapter 6:

EVALUATION AND DIAGNOSIS OF ERECTILE DYSFUNCTION (ED)

Your healthcare provider will take a sexual history. Data includes how the Erectile Dysfunction developed, if you have morning erections or not, any interpersonal problems with a sexual partner, and any risk factors such as history of smoking, diabetes, high cholesterol, depression, high blood pressure, and alcohol usage. If symptoms last more than three months, it is pertinent and needs to be treated. The earlier the treatment, the greater the chance of improvement or resolution.

A physical exam is performed to check your pulse for any abnormal swelling in the extremities and to check the penis and scrotum for any masses, curvature, scars, or pain to palpation. A digital prostate exam is expected.

The provider may order serum blood tests for hormones such as testosterone, prolactin, and thyroid hormones. Elevated prolactin and low testosterone and low or high levels of thyroid hormone can contribute to sexual dysfunction.

Sometimes, a more specialized test, such as a penile color Doppler ultrasound, will be done during a pharmacologically-induced erection to assess arterial and venous flow in the penis.

It is essential that the patient answers all questions accurately and provides as much detail as possible during this evaluation. The more details you provide the doctor, the better your treatment outcome.

Erectile function can be measured using the International Index of Erectile Function (IIEF). Men with risk factors for ED and scores of less than 25 on the IIEF may benefit from sildenafil and the Priapus Shot®.

INTERNATIONAL INDEX OF ERECTILE DYSFUNCTION (IIEF)

INSTRUCTIONS: These questions ask about your sex life over the past four weeks. Please answer the following questions as honestly and clearly as possible. In answering these questions, the following definitions apply:

Sexual activity includes intercourse, caressing, foreplay, and masturbation.

Sexual intercourse is defined as vaginal penetration of the partner (you entered your partner).

Sexual stimulation includes situations like foreplay with a partner, looking at erotic pictures, etc.

Ejaculate refers to the ejection of semen from the penis (or the feeling of this).

1. Over the past four weeks, how often were you able to get an erection during sexual activity?

0 = No sexual activity

1 = Almost never or never

2 = A few times (much less than half the time)

3 = Sometimes (about half the time)

4 = Most times (much more than half the time)

5 = Almost always or always

2. Over the past four weeks, when you had erections with sexual stimulation, how often were your erections hard enough for penetration?

0 = No sexual activity

1 = Almost never or never

2 = A few times (much less than half the time)

3 = Sometimes (about half the time)

4 = Most times (much more than half the time)

5 = Almost always or always

The next eight questions will ask about the erections you may have had during sexual intercourse.

3. Over the past four weeks, when you attempted sexual intercourse, how often were you able to penetrate (enter) your partner?

0 = Did not attempt intercourse

1 = Almost never or never

2 = A few times (much less than half the time)

3 = Sometimes (about half the time)

4 = Most times (much more than half the time)

5 = Almost always or always

4. Over the past four weeks, during sexual intercourse, how often were you able to maintain your erection after you penetrated (entered) your partner?

0 = Did not attempt intercourse

1 = Almost never or never

2 = A few times (much less than half the time)

3 = Sometimes (about half the time)

4 = Most times (much more than half the time)

5 = Almost always or always

5. Over the past four weeks, during sexual intercourse, how difficult was it to maintain your erection to completion of intercourse?

0 = Did not attempt intercourse

1 = Extremely difficult

2 = Very difficult

3 = Difficult

4 = Slightly difficult

5 = Not difficult

6. Over the past four weeks, how many times have you attempted sexual intercourse?

0 = No attempts

1 = One to two attempts

2 = Three to four attempts

3 = Five to six attempts

4 = 7 to 10 attempts

5 = 11 or more attempts

7. Over the past four weeks, when you attempted sexual intercourse, how often was it satisfactory for you?

0 = Did not attempt intercourse

1 = Almost never or never

2 = A few times (much less than half the time)

3 = Sometimes (about half the time)

4 = Most times (much more than half the time)

5 = Almost always or always

8. Over the past four weeks, when you attempted sexual intercourse, how much have you enjoyed sexual intercourse?

0 = No intercourse

1 = No enjoyment

2 = Not very enjoyable

3 = Fairly enjoyable

4 = Highly enjoyable

5 = Very highly enjoyable

9. Over the past four weeks, when you had sexual stimulation or intercourse, how often did you ejaculate?

0 = No sexual stimulation/intercourse

1 = Almost never or never

2 = A few times (much less than half the time)

3 = Sometimes (about half the time)

4 = Most times (much more than half the time)

5 = Almost always or always

10. Over the past four weeks, when you had sexual stimulation or intercourse, how often did you have the feeling of orgasm or climax?

0 = No sexual stimulation/intercourse

1 = Almost never or never

2 = A few times (much less than half the time)

3 = Sometimes (about half the time)

4 = Most times (much more than half the time)

5 = Almost always or always

The next five questions ask about sexual desire. Sexual desire as a feeling that may include wanting to have a sexual experience (for example, masturbation or intercourse), thinking about having sex, or feeling frustrated due to lack of sex.

11. Over the past four weeks, how often have you felt sexual desire?

1 = Almost never or never

2 = A few times (much less than half the time)

3 = Sometimes (about half the time)

4 = Most times (much more than half the time)

5 = Almost always or always

12. Over the past four weeks, how would you rate your level of sexual desire?

1 = Very low or not at all

2 = Low

3 = Moderate

4 = High

5 = Very high

13. Over the past four weeks, how satisfied have you been with your overall sex life?

1 = Very dissatisfied

2 = Moderately dissatisfied

3 = About equally satisfied and dissatisfied

4 = Moderately satisfied

5 = Very satisfied

14. Over the past four weeks, how satisfied have you been with your sexual relationship with your partner?

1 = Very dissatisfied

2 = Moderately dissatisfied

3 = About equally satisfied and dissatisfied

4 = Moderately satisfied

5 = Very satisfied

15. Over the past four weeks, how do you rate your confidence that you can get and keep an erection?

1 = Very low

2 = Low

3 = Moderate

4 = High

5 = Very high

Rosen RC, Riley A, Wagner G, et al. The International index of Erectile Dysfunction (IIEF): a multidimensional scale for assessment of erectile dysfunction. Urology 1997; 49:822. Illustration used with the permission of Elsevier Inc. All rights reserved.

Chapter 7:

TREATMENTS FOR ERECTILE DYSFUNCTION

Erectile Dysfunction is very common, yet a man may not know there are solutions available. Or the man is embarrassed to ask his doctor or friends. He may suffer in silence. There are choices other than medications and surgery. Knowing the existing treatment options for ED makes it tolerable and perhaps treatable.

Drugs for Erectile Dysfunction:

Medications such as phosphodiesterase-5 inhibitors: sildenafil (Viagra), vardenafil (Levitra), tadalafil (Cialis), and avanafil (Stendra), are all phosphodiesterase (PDE-5) inhibitors. They have restored potency efficiently in 70% of men. They work better in men with psychogenic impotence. All four PDE-5 inhibitors enhance intracavernosal (intra-penile tissues) cyclic guanosine monophosphate (GMP) levels. Cyclic GMP elevates nitric oxide levels to improve the erectile response to sexual stimulation in many men with ED.

However, these medications are contraindicated in men on nitrates, a medication for angina. Nitrates should not be used within 48 hours after the last dose of erectile enhancement drug use. Alpha blockers are medications used for hypertension and benign prostatic hypertrophy. These drugs include terazosin, doxazosin, tamsulosin, alfuzosin, and silodosin. These medications can cause hypotension and impaired ejaculations when used with phosphodiesterase -5 inhibitors.

Medications have to be taken on an empty stomach and can last 6-24 hours. Another inconvenience is that there is no spontaneity, and sexual activity must be planned 30 minutes to 1 hour ahead. Eating a fatty meal before Viagra and Levitra can reduce the effectiveness of the drug. Wait 2-3 hours after eating before taking these medications.

Common Side Effects of PDE- 5 inhibitors:

- Headache
- Flushing in the face, neck, or chest
- Upset stomach, indigestion
- Abnormal vision, "blue vision"
- Nasal congestion
- Back pain

- Muscular pain or tenderness
- Nausea
- Dizziness
- Rash
- Diarrhea

Serious Side Effects of PDE-5 inhibitors:

- Change or loss of vision
- Ringing in ears or hearing loss
- Chest pain or irregular heartbeat
- Shortness of breath
- Lightheadedness
- Swelling of the hands, ankles, and feet
- Pulmonary hypertension
- Malignant melanoma

PDE-5 inhibitors have many other severe interactions with other commonly used drugs. It is recommended that you discuss this with your doctor before and during the use of this class of drugs. Your doctor will counsel if it is safe to use with other drugs. Sildenafil (Viagra) is associated with a short duration of post-ejaculatory refractory time, or a short time frame until next erection. Thus, recreational use of sildenafil is common.

Penile Self Injection:

Less commonly used drug options include prostaglandin E1, such as alprostadil and papaverine for inducing erection by injection into the cavernosum tissues. This class of drug opens arteries, resulting in improvement of an erection.

Phentolamine is added to papaverine to make a compound called BiMix. If a prostaglandin E1 is added, it is called TriMix. TriMix is injected into the penis to stimulate an erection. However, penile injections are at risk for plaque development. Often, this is discontinued due to penile pain. Priapism, an erection lasting longer than 4-6 hours, is a complication and needs emergency treatment. Prolonged priapism results in penile fibrosis and exacerbated erectile dysfunction as a consequence.

A prostaglandin E1, alprostadil, can be injected into the urethra followed by a massage for up to 1 min. It is less effective than the penile injection and has complications of pain and bleeding.

Low-Intensity Shockwave Therapy:

Low-Intensity Shockwave therapy is not new. It has been used in cardiology, diabetic assessment, and urology. Low-intensity shockwave therapy for sexual medicine is a novelty and is an emerging innovation for non-pharmacological therapy treatment for erectile dysfunction.

Multiple studies are now showing results with improvement on the Erectile Dysfunction scale (IIEF) after low-intensity shock-wave therapy. This treatment improved blood flow to the penis [30] for men with erectile dysfunction from blood flow impairments.

Shockwave therapy uses energy from acoustic waves to trigger a process called neovascularization in certain parts of the body. Neovascularization occurs when tissues undergo microtrauma from the shock waves. When neovascularization occurs, new blood vessels form. New blood vessels help improve blood flow to the penis.

This type of therapy has been used to help heart patients, people with kidney stones, and those with fractures and joint inflammation.

This treatment involves a handheld probe device held to the penis to deliver low shock waves. The treatment feels like someone tapping with their finger on the penis. Pain control is not needed; however, sometimes a numbing cream is placed on the penis before the procedure for more comfort. Five regions of the penis are treated, and this procedure only takes 20 minutes.

After the procedure, improvement in IIEF scores and improvement in Erectile Dysfunction is sustained at a year. Low-intensity shock wave treats the source of the problem with blood flow in ED. In conjunction with the Priapus Shot®, the effects will be longer lasting.

Low-intensity shockwave therapy treatment alone may convert men not responding to PDE-5 inhibitors to responders.

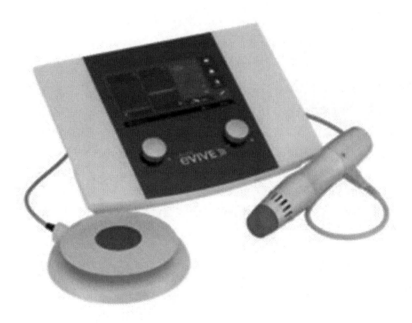

Low-Intensity Shock Wave Machine

The Pump Theory:

The vacuum pump is a low-cost and reasonable treatment for erectile dysfunction. The vacuum pumps have also proved successful in studies of penile rehabilitation. Radical prostatectomies can cause temporary impotence as a result of nerve damage. If you go long enough without a spontaneous erection, some of your penile tissue can atrophy, causing long-term dysfunction. Most often, postoperative use of a penis pump may help stave off this damage. Penis pumps are available over the counter.

The device consists of an acrylic tube and a pumping mechanism, which can be a manual or electric device. As the user pumps air out of the tube, the resulting vacuum increases blood flow into his erectile tissue. A "constriction ring" slides over the base of his penis to maintain the erection when he removes the tube.

As explained by Dr. Charles Runels: An erection can be modeled as a water balloon. A balloon grows to a size where the inside pressure equals the outside pressure. A balloon with no air pressure collapses because there's no pressure on the inside to make it expand to match atmospheric pressure. When you blow into the balloon, then the balloon expands to a point where the inside pressure matches the tension or elasticity of the wall of the balloon. When you blow up a balloon, you can feel that tension and that it limits the size of the balloon; you can also feel that it's the tension in the wall that makes it difficult to blow up the balloon.

To decrease the forces that contract the penis is to decrease the penile tissue tension.

Here are four reasons for using the pump:

- To raise penile oxygen levels; the flaccid penis has lower oxygen saturation that other parts of the body.
- To avoid contraction.
- To stretch out the bent places that occur with conditions like Peyronie's.
- To get an erection with the pump, thereby bringing more oxygen to the tissue. Research (39) showed that men who use a penis pump daily feed their penis oxygen.

Using the pump too frequently with too much pressure can cause scar tissue. You should use the pump and the P Shot®.

Other side effects of the penis pump are darkened skin, swelling post pump removal, and pain.

Another interesting phenomenon is decreased the function of the penis. The phenomenon is called "turtling." It is when the penis may feel rubbery, or puffy, and seems tired. To improve this, give the penis a rest.

Don't use the pump for a week. Avoid ejaculation for two weeks. Let your penis recover.

Your best penis and your best mental, physical, and spiritual health are all going to be achieved when you consider the whole picture.

The pump and the P Shot® work together like light weight lifting and anabolic steroids. Together they will give you your best penis and will coincide with good mental, physical, and spiritual health to complete you as a whole person.

The thing that differs about both of these treatments, versus what we have had available (for example, Viagra or injecting a vasodilator), is that neither of those two things corrects the problem. With the Priapus Shot®, we're getting to the etiology.

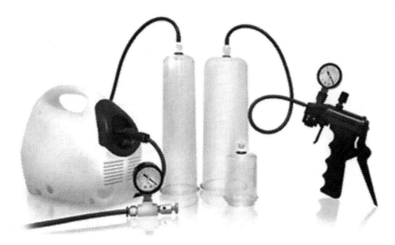

Electric and manual vacuum pumps

Testosterone Therapy:

With age, a man's total testosterone level decreases from age 40-79 by 0.4% a year (70). Young men have a high testosterone level at 8 am and 8 pm, whereas older men have a steady testosterone level throughout the day.

This decline is called andropause or late-onset hypogonadism. This fall might have consequences in energy, sexual function, muscle mass, red blood cells, and bone density. The decline may lead to obesity and other conditions such as diabetes mellitus.

Testosterone plays an essential role in male sexual function. Testosterone Deficiency (TD) is an important condition that can profoundly affect men. Testosterone Deficiency, also known as hypogonadism, is a common medical condition affecting men, and is characterized by signs and symptoms of low testosterone as well as decreased serum testosterone level.

Testosterone Deficiency results in impotence in animal and human experimentation and sexual potency returns when testosterone levels are normalized [8]. Testosterone works through psychogenic channels to enhance libido. Furthermore, testosterone maintains nitric oxide synthase (i.e. makes nitric oxide for erection) activity.

Testosterone Effects:

- Enhance libido
- Sexual desire
- Erection, morning erection
- Maintenance of intrapenile nitric oxide synthase levels, maintain an erection
- Maintain bone mineral density and prevent fractures
- Maintain Muscle and decrease fat mass
- Maintain muscle strength
- Prevents anemia
- Improves mood, energy
- Improves cognitive function
- Metabolic, cardiovascular protection: resists central obesity and insulin resistance protects against metabolic syndrome, diabetes, high sensitivity C-reactive protein.

Symptoms of Testosterone Deficiency:

- Sexual
  - ❖ Decreased sexual desire and activity
  - ❖ Decreased frequency of sexual thoughts
  - ❖ Decreased frequency of morning erections
  - ❖ Erectile dysfunction

- ❖ Delayed ejaculation
- ❖ A small volume of ejaculation
- Physical
  - ❖ Inability to perform vigorous activity
  - ❖ Decreased physical vigor and muscle strength
  - ❖ Decreased ability to bend
  - ❖ Fatigue
  - ❖ Hot flashes and sweats
- Psychological
  - ❖ Decreased energy, motivation, initiative
  - ❖ Depressed mood
  - ❖ Sadness
  - ❖ Excessive irritability
  - ❖ Sleep disturbances, insomnia, sleepiness
  - ❖ Poor self- rated health
- Cognitive
  - ❖ Impaired concentration
  - ❖ Impaired verbal memory
  - ❖ Impair spatial performance

Testosterone Deficiency can result from either low testosterone secretion from the pituitary gland in the brain or from the testicles. It can also be low due to impaired androgen receptor function or the blockage of the androgen receptor or increased sex hormone binding globulin, which can result in decreased free testosterone or bioavailable testosterone.

Testosterone Deficiency is a clinical symptom of low testosterone and characterized by laboratory findings of low testosterone. Testosterone Deficiency is defined by the presence of three symptoms of low testosterone with a total testosterone level lower than 320 ng/dL (11 nmol/L), and a free testosterone level lower than 6.4 ng/dL (6.4 pg/mL, 220 pmol/L).

Erectile Dysfunction is associated with a lower testosterone level of 350 ng/dL. It is recommended that men with Erectile Dysfunction be tested for total testosterone level and to be checked to see if their serum level is low. Testosterone Deficiency should be treated as an adjunct to the P Shot® for Erectile Dysfunction.

Low testosterone is often associated in men with chronic diseases:

- Concussion
- Obesity
- Type 2 diabetes
- Metabolic syndrome
- Coronary artery disease
- Hypertension
- COPD
- Osteoporosis

- Chronic heart disease
- Atrial fibrillation
- Heart failure
- Cirrhosis
- Rheumatoid arthritis
- Cancer
- Chronic opioid use
- End-stage renal disease

Men with these chronic conditions are recommended for low testosterone screening.

Testosterone therapy was associated with a moderate improvement in sexual function in men with low libido, including sexual activity, sexual desire (libido), and erectile function. The magnitude of the rise in serum testosterone and estradiol concentrations were associated with the magnitude of improvement in sexual desire and sexual activity, but not erectile function [7]. Erectile Dysfunction involves more than just testosterone alone, but a combination of a medical conditions as discussed previously.

There is no compelling evidence that testosterone treatment increases the risk of developing prostate cancer or the progression of prostate cancer. [8,9].

The data on cardiac complications, such as heart attacks and strokes, associated with testosterone therapy have been conflicting. The Food and Drug Administration (FDA) issued a Safety Announcement in 2015 requiring manufacturers of testosterone products to include warnings concerning the possible increased risk of cardiac complications.

Testosterone therapy has different formulations. Testosterone can be given as troche, as a transdermal gel, in subcutaneous pellets, or an intramuscular injection. Follow-up testosterone screenings should be completed every 3-6 months.

Chapter 8:

LIFESTYLE CHANGES TO IMPROVE ERECTILE DYSFUNCTION

LIFESTYLE CHANGES:

Lifestyle changes should be the first treatment option to consider for Erectile Dysfunction. Weight loss and physical activity have been correlated with better sexual function, compared to men who are obese and do not perform physical activity. Gastric bypass patients have been shown to improve testosterone levels and erectile function, as well as well as show a decrease in sleep apnea. Modifying risk factors for cardiovascular disease (high blood pressure, high cholesterol, and diabetes) by weight loss can lead to better sexual function.

Stopping smoking and alcohol can also be beneficial for sexual function. Instead of taking medication for high blood pressure or pain, it may be useful to consider weight reduction as a way to improve libido.

Exercises for Erectile Dysfunction:

The best way to treat Erectile Dysfunction without medication is by strengthening the pelvic floor muscles with Kegel exercises, along with lifestyle changes. Kegel exercises are often associated with women looking to strengthen their pelvic area post-pregnancy, but they can be useful for men looking to regain full function of the penis.

Pelvic floor muscle activation can be achieved by stopping mid-stream two or three times when you urinate. The muscles you can feel working during this process are the pelvic floor muscles, and they will be the focus of Kegel exercises.

One Kegel exercise consists of tightening and holding these muscles for 5 seconds and then releasing them. Try to do between 10 and 20 repetitions each day. Holding for 20 seconds may not be possible when you first start doing the exercises. However, they should become easier over time. Improvement is noted after six weeks.

Make sure you are breathing naturally throughout this process and avoid pushing down as if you are forcing urination. Instead, bring the muscles together in a squeezing motion upward towards your belly button but avoid squeezing your buttocks muscles the same time.

It is suggested that you see a physical or occupational therapist specializing in pelvic floor therapy to assist with proper Kegel exercises, as these exercises can often be performed incorrectly. Kegel exercises must be coordinated with inspiration and expiration. Improper coordination can result in the worsening of pelvic floor muscle strength.

Because erectile dysfunction is caused by decreased blood flow to the penis, aerobic exercise, such as a jog or even a brisk walk, can also help the blood to circulate better and can help improve ED in men who have circulation issues.

Chapter 9:

SURGICAL TREATMENT FOR ERECTILE DYSFUNCTION

Men with significant cardiovascular disease are not good candidates for penile revascularization; however, if their cardiac risk is not high, they may be a candidate for a penile implant.

A significant advance in prosthetic surgery has been the placement of devices within the paired corpora cavernosa, providing improved cosmetic and functional results [10, 11, 12].

There are several surgical treatment options:

- <u>Penile implants</u>: These are a final option reserved for men who have not had any success with drug treatments and other non-invasive options.

  Two types of penile implants are commercially available, with inflatable prosthetics accounting for the majority of implants [14].

Implant infection occurs in approximately 3% of cases; patients with diabetes, spinal cord injury, or previous implants have infection rates up to 10 percent [17,18,].

- Semi-rigid: They are easy to use but result in a permanent erection. Semi-rigid make up less than 10% of all implanted penile prostheses [15].

- Malleable devices: They are excellent and are accessible to implant. Because they are malleable, the penis can be bent down close to the body to be less noticeable under clothing.

- Inflatable: The inflatable prostheses are designed to approximate the rigidity and flaccidity of the normally functioning penis. These devices consist of two hollow cylinders placed within the corpora cavernosa, a saline reservoir and pump [16].

- Vascular surgery: Another surgical option for some men is vascular surgery, which attempts to correct some causes of ED involving the blood vessels. Postoperative complications may include penile edema, penile numbness, and penile shortening due to scar entrapment. Only 6-7% of men with vascular erectile dysfunction are candidates for penile revascularization [19]. Long-term success rates range from 50-67% [19, 20, 21, 22].

Surgery is a last resort and will only be used in the most extreme cases.

Chapter 10:

WHAT IS PLATELET RICH PLASMA (PRP)?

Platelet Rich Plasma or PRP is a preparation of your blood into a platelet concentrate in a smaller volume after processing in the centrifuge. PRP is prepared by centrifuging autologous and anticoagulated whole blood to separate its component and concentrate platelets above baseline. Typically, 30 cc or 60 cc of blood is taken out from the vein in the arm and deposited in an FDA approved kit and then centrifuged. After a few minutes, the kit chamber separates the whole blood into the top plasma layer, the middle layer of leukocytes (white blood cells) layer and a bottom red blood cell layer. The process takes between 5-15 minutes, depending on the device. Components of PRP include platelets, which contain growth factors, leukocytes, and red blood cells.

PRP has vital regenerative growth factors stored in the platelets granules [31, 32, 33, 34]:

- EGF – Endothelial Growth Factor
  - ❖ Induce cell growth and tensile strength
- IGF1 – Insulin-like Growth Factor
  - ❖ Regulates cell growth and differentiation
  - ❖ Influences collagen and noncollagenous proteins
- VEGF – Vascular Endothelial Growth Factor
  - ❖ Stimulates new blood vessel growth
- PDGF – Platelet Derived Growth Factor
  - ❖ Stimulates cell growth and new blood vessels
- bFGF – Basic Fibroblast Growth Factor
  - ❖ Stimulates new blood vessels
  - ❖ Promotes stem cell differentiation and cell growth
  - ❖ Promotes collagen production and repairs tissue
- TGF – Beta – Transforming Growth Factor – Beta
  - ❖ Stimulates collagen type I, III
  - ❖ Stimulates new blood vessels
  - ❖ Inhibit collagen breakdown

PRP supplies and release growth factors from the platelets to stimulate a regenerative response that augments healing and promotes repair in tissues that would not normally happen in tissues with injury or low healing potential.

PRP has been used in chronic wound medicine for a long time, and its regenerative potential was realized in the 1980's and 1990's with applications in cardiac surgery, dental, and maxillary facial surgery. PRP is used today in skeletal muscle medicine due to its potential for healing. PRP can heal soft tissues and muscles, and this has translated to aesthetic and sexual medicine.

PRP is used to promote healing in soft tissue (such as muscle tendon, ligament, and cartilage), which has slow and inadequate potential for healing due to the limited blood supply and slow cell turnover. PRP essentially stimulates wound healing by inflammation, proliferation and remodeling of soft tissue. The inflammation stage is from day 0 to day 6. The proliferation stage is from day 6 to day 14, and the maturation and proliferation stage is from day 8 to 1 year but peaking at three months. Different structures of the body heal at different rates.

Factors that affect healing include decreased oxygen due to cardiac dysfunction, peripheral vascular disease, systemic diseases such as connective tissue disorder or diabetes mellitus, hypothyroidism, malignancy organ failure, connective tissue disorders such as Ehlers-Danlos syndrome, and osteogenesis imperfecta.

Nutrition plays a critical role in protein synthesis, as muscle is primarily made up of proteins. Muscle is essential in the healing process, and healing needs collagen. Vitamin A, C and D, zinc, copper, and iron are important in immune function and healing.

Also, smoking and alcohol can impair tissue repair. Nonsteroidal anti-inflammatory drugs distressed the connective tissue healing cascade in animal studies. Corticosteroids or cortisone affect healing pathways by decreasing immune response.

Soft tissue healing cascade with Platelet Rich Plasma:

After the PRP is injected, the platelet granules burst into the tissue and growth factors are released immediately. These growth factors cause white blood cells to create an inflammation from the time of injection until 3-5 days after. Cell growth starts on day 1 until day 21 and peaks at day 10. A remodeling phase or collagen restructuring starts around day 11, peaks at 42 days, and continues until 100 days or more.

PRP can work synergistically with stem cells from the bone marrow called Hematopoietic stem cells and with adipose (fat) stem cells called mesenchymal stem cells to regenerate joints (knees, hips, shoulders, ankles), the spine, muscles, and tendons. Stem cells and PRP therapies offer healing, pain-free living for any age. PRP is the most effective treatment and should be considered as first-line therapy.

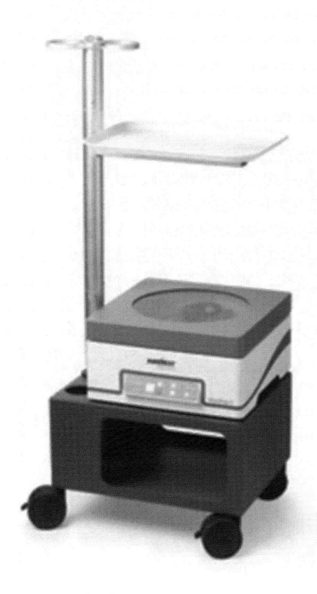

Platelet Rich Plasma Centrifuge

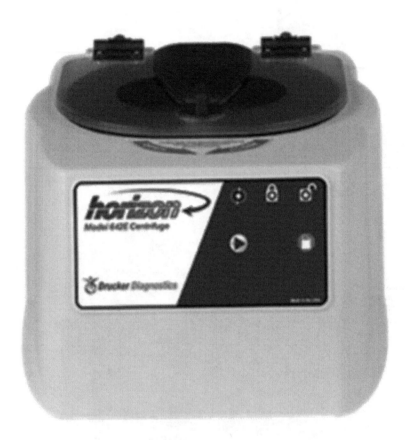

Platelet Rich Plasma Centrifuge

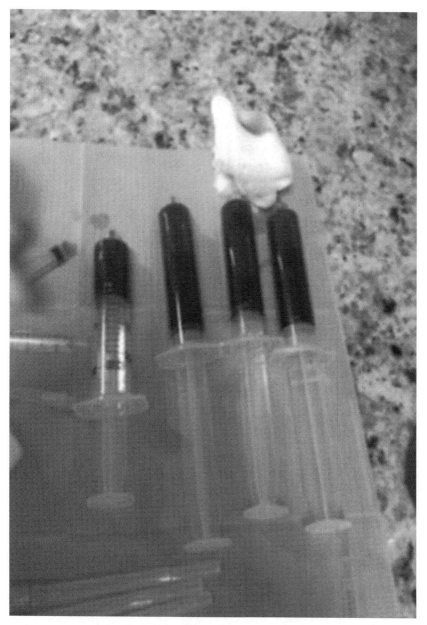

Blood drawn from veins into syringes

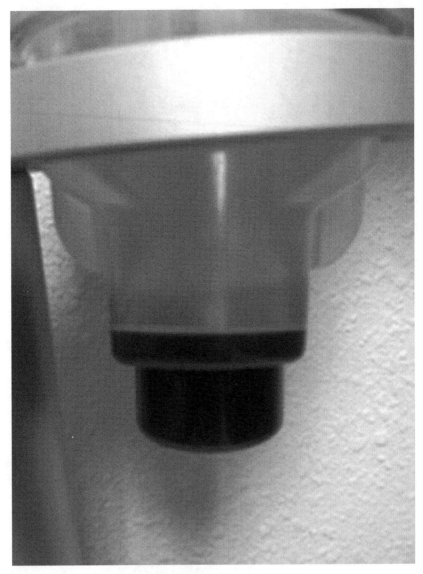

Platelets Rich Plasma (PRP)

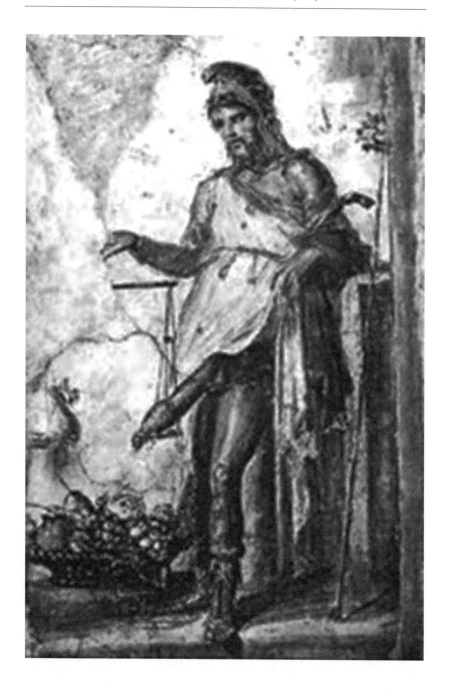

Chapter 11:

THE PRIAPUS SHOT®
(P-SHOT®)

The Priapus Shot® is the natural solution to treat Erectile Dysfunction. Viagra and medications like it, penile implants, penile injectables, and hormones do not create new blood vessels to the penis.

How does Platelet Rich Plasma (PRP) work for Erectile Dysfunction?

PRP, when injected into an injured area, can regenerate the tissue by increasing blood flow and regenerating cell proliferation. When PRP is injected into the penis and the glans, over a period of weeks to months, it creates new vascular proliferation and new soft tissue to improve vascular flow to the penis and therefore improves the ability to maintain an erection.

The Priapus Shot® or P Shot® is an injection of concentrated platelets into the penis. The penis is prepared by applying a numbing topical cream. The PRP is processed in an FDA approved kit that processes whole blood which is drawn up from a vein. The whole blood is placed into the kit, and the kit is put in a centrifuge. After a few minutes, the blood is separated into a Platelet Rich layer. This is drawn up into a syringe and is then injected painlessly into the penis.

The preparation of the PRP involves a device approved by the FDA for isolating PRP from whole blood for autologous use. Since blood is not a drug, it is not governed by the FDA, but the FDA regulates the devices used to isolate PRP for injection back into the body. Multiple kits have gained FDA approval. Some of the approved kits include Regen, Magellan, TruPRP, Eclipse, Pure Spin, Harvest, and Emcyte. There are over 8,000 research papers in multiple journals discussing the science of PRP, and not one serious side effect has been documented when FDA approved kits were used to prepare the PRP.

A very small needle (1/2-inch-long, 30 gauge) is used for the injection. However, some men do ask for a dorsal nerve block, which can quickly be done using 2% lidocaine for a near painless procedure (this same block can be used for prosthesis placement—so it makes a 30-gauge needle entirely painless for most men).

The Priapus Shot® shows improvement in the health, circulation, and strength (density) of penile tissue due to the injection of blood-derived growth factors into the penis.

The procedure takes no more than 10 minutes. The patient does not feel pain, just pressure. There is no downtime for this procedure. The patient will feel the penis is engorged for about 1-3 days, but then any swelling will go down. The patient can have sex the night of the procedure.

It is recommended that he uses a penis pump after the procedure. The patient will have peak sensation and a suitable correction by three weeks that will last until nine months to a year. Some patients may require more than one shot. With each subsequent shot, he will become more sensitive, have a firmer erection, and have a better and more intense orgasm. This painless procedure can improve sex, libido, and relationships.

There are no side effects other than some slight bruising. It does cause penis engorgement initially and may create a 10% improvement in girth and width.

Patients will be selected very carefully depending on co-morbidities present. If the patient has vascular problems, such as coronary artery disease, high blood pressure, diabetes, or peripheral vascular disease, they may have slow healing and may need more than one P Shot®.

Who does the Priapus Shot® (P-Shot®) not benefit?

Nothing is perfect: There is no perfect procedure and some patients simply are not candidates. Men suffering from psychological abuse or another psychological component would not be appropriate for this procedure. After the procedure, the result is better with adequate testosterone supplementation, along with the penile pump and healthy lifestyle behavior. This person will, more likely than not have better results versus someone who just gets the P Shot® alone without evaluation of hormonal needs.

A patient may have difficulty responding if the patient does not respond to Viagra or has severe vascular disease, pituitary hormonal dysfunction, or structural problems proximal to the penis.

Medical insurance does not cover the P Shot® at this time. The procedure was created in 2014 by Dr. Charles Runels, and it will likely take about 20 years or so for insurance to approve this as an alternative.

The Priapus Shot® is a new way to use blood-derived growth factors to rehabilitate the penis.

What Goes with the Shot?

For improvement in erection firmness, the Priapus Shot® protocol also includes a recommendation of aerobic exercise and use of the penis pump. Both have been effective with the P Shot® as part of an effective penile rehabilitation program.

Dr. Virag's studies, using the injection of PRP as a stand-alone (without physical therapies), also demonstrated improvement in the angle of the penis in men suffering from Peyronie's disease [23].

Also, strict adherence to a penis pump regimen is part of the Priapus Shot® protocol, and the pump alone improves the angle significantly in over one-half of patients in one study in the British Journal of Urology [26]. This same study demonstrated the growth of the penis using the pump alone (without the PRP injection). The PRP alone, in Dr. Virag's study, out-performed the pump with a demonstration of remodeling of the plaque. The vacuum pump and the Priapus Shot® are recommended for treatment of Peyronie's disease.

Studies show that the non-surgical treatment of Peyronie's is most effective when a synergy of multiple modalities is engaged [27]. The Priapus Shot® procedure includes the injection of PRP combined with daily physical therapy using a penis pump for ten minutes, twice a day and a daily low-dose of tadalafil. Such strategies are not intended to take the place of surgical correction or the use of chemical surgery with collagenase—but rather to offer the man suffering from Peyronie's disease the optimal non-surgical treatment as a first step, with surgery reserved if non-surgical therapies fail.

The penis pump alone (part of the Priapus Shot® protocol) has been shown to improve the effectiveness of Cialis and Trimix injections [28]. We are seeing men decrease the dosage of Viagra and Trimix by about 50 percent when the complete Priapus Shot® protocol is used. The Priapus Shot® protocol does not intend to make any particular therapy obsolete (including surgery), but rather to offer a protocol for enhancing an overall, synergistic approach to correcting penile pathology.

However, the surgical treatment of Peyronie's disease can be unsatisfying and lead to serious complications [29]. The Priapus Shot® protocol offers an appealing, conservative, and often effective step to take before proceeding to surgery. The risk from PRP is undoubtedly much less than for surgery and less than for collagenase—offering another reason to start with the Priapus Shot® when treating Peyronie's Disease or Erectile Dysfunction.

In over 8,000 papers published about PRP, there is not one serious sequela reported. It seems logical when you consider the material being injected is autologous (your own tissues) and customarily produced to heal and to fight infection.

Stem cells are not directly prepared as part of the Priapus Shot® procedure. PRP hones the stem cells from the body to the injection site. These stem cells accelerate the healing process.

The idea of safety is further emphasized by the literature indicating that not only are there no reports of severe allergic reactions to PRP, but PRP can attenuate the autoimmune response. This attribute of PRP could partly explain the effectiveness of the Priapus Shot® protocol for the treatment of both Peyronie's Disease and Erectile Dysfunction, since Peyronie's Disease is thought to be partly caused by an autoimmune response.

Our provider's group observed that only 60% of men achieve 1/2 inch or more in penis growth (circumference and length). But, men in that 60% sometimes see up to 1.5 inches in circumference and length (often after 2 to 3 procedures one month apart).

Men with long-standing vascular disease have less improvement. If the blood flow going to the penis (iliac arteries) is blocked, then the Priapus Shot® injection into the penis will not help much. The patient needs a vascular surgeon. For example, if the patient sees no response when taking Viagra or Cialis for more than two years, then he may have blockages or other problems that the Priapus Shot® will not help.

P Shot® can be used for postoperative penile rehabilitation for prostate surgery. If the man could achieve erection before the surgery, then following the Priapus Shot® protocol could be very beneficial (even if it has been 2 or 3 years since surgery).

With the Priapus Shot®, an improved firmness of erection can be achieved. It is typical that the patient may be able to cut the dose of Viagra or Trimix in half (but still need the drug), or if he needs only a low dose of the drugs, he may be able to stop using them.

Lichen Sclerosis appears on the foreskin with severe discomfort and often recurs even if the man has a circumcision. The P Shot® can improve Lichen Sclerosis.

The Priapus Shot® can improve Peyronie's Disease. It is safer and more effective than collagenase injections. If a man undergoes surgery for Peyronie's Disease, the curvature often recurs later since the autoimmune process continues. Also, with surgery, there can be infection and shortening of the penis. None of these side effects have been seen with the Priapus Shot® procedure. In fact, the opposite occurs in most patients with Peyronie's disease witnessing an increase in size.

SUMMARY OF THE PRIAPUS SHOT®

In summary, multiple studies support the idea that blood-derived growth factors (when prepared in a proper way using a kit approved by the FDA for the preparation of PRP), as used in the Priapus Shot® protocol, support the health and function of the penis. Erectile Dysfunction is associated with anhedonia (a general lack of pleasure), and successful treatment leads to better function, better relationships, and more pleasure in life[27].

The Priapus Shot® procedure indicates a specific way of treating the penis with blood-derived growth factors extracted from the man's own blood (autologous). Some people call these blood-derived growth factors Platelet-Rich Plasma (PRP), but there may be growth factors in plasma we don't yet know about that do not come from the platelets. The name "Priapus Shot®" is registered with the US Patent & Trademark Office as a "service mark" to protect patients by indicating a specific protocol. The name is not a synonym for the injection of blood into the penis—such a definition would not be accurate enough to indicate any particular quality of care-- so it would not warrant protection as intellectual property.

Dr. Virag (also a pioneer of Trimix injections) published research demonstrating improvement in erectile function, size, and correction of Peyronie's disease with the use of PRP. His past and future studies show a mean increase of 7 on the ED Intensity Score when PRP is injected into the plaque and the corpus cavernosum of the human penis [23].

The trademark defines a specific method that providers agree to follow and develop. Currently, around the world, there are 1,518 providers of various specialties who perform the P Shot®.

Benefits of the Priapus Shot®:

- Immediately larger for three days
- For enlargement, for a longer time, the protocol involved doing the injections once a month for five injections total and to use the penis pump for 20 minutes every day for three months.
- Strengthening of the penis
- Straightening of the penis
- Increased circulation within the penis for a healthier organ.
- Other therapies will work better (if you still need Viagra or Cialis, then it will work better for you).
- Increased sensation and pleasure (helps correct the damage from diabetes).
- Proven to work in multiple studies
- Increased size by design (Can place more in the base or the head or wherever makes for best result)
- No allergic reactions (using your blood).
- No lumpiness
- Minimal pain
- Helps with Lichens Sclerosis
- Helps with Peyronie's Disease

To get the best result for Erectile Dysfunction, see a health care provider for evaluation and diagnoses. The

Priapus Shot® should be the first line of therapy. Along with optimizing hormones, lifestyle changes are encouraged to address the problem as a whole.

Men should not suffer from Erectile Dysfunction anymore; there is a solution with the Priapus Shot®, and it will change lives.

To find a health care provider who can perform the Priapus Shot protocol, go www.priapusshot.com/members/directory .

Chapter 12:

OTHER BENEFITS OF PLATELET RICH PLASMA

It is an exciting era for regenerative medicine. Research on Platelet Rich Plasma (PRP) continues to show advancement and improvement in orthopedic and soft tissue healing.

Aside from soft tissue healing from aesthetic and sexuality conditions, PRP therapy indication also includes:

- Chronic pain and arthritis pain from the knee, ankle, shoulder, and hip
- Ligament injury: Ankle, plantar fascia, sacroiliac joint, knee, and hip
- Tendon injury: Medial and lateral epicondylitis, rotator cuff injury, hip tendinitis, and ankle tendinitis
- Acute and chronic muscle tears

There are contraindications to Platelet Rich Plasma (PRP) therapy:

#1 Active infection

#2 Immunocompromised status

#3 Blood clotting disorders or an INR greater than 2.5

#4 Pain in the prosthetic joint or infection

PRP can be used in conjunction with bone marrow stem cells and adipose stem cells to treat more advanced injuries and arthritis cases. Stem cells from bone marrow and fat can replenish dying cells and regenerate damaged tissues. These stem cells are called mesenchymal stem cells. They have the potential to differentiate into a variety of tissues such as bone, cartilage, fat, muscle, tendon, and ligament. These mesenchymal stem cells are involved in the development and repair of bone and cartilage. Orthopedic surgeons have been using cancellous bone chips to assist in the repair of nonunion fractures since the 1930's.

Several innovative FDA approved kits physicians can use to harvest mesenchymal cells from bone marrow is the MARROW CELLUTION™ bone marrow trocar. MARROW CELLUTION™ maximizes hematopoietic stem cell recovery while minimizing peripheral blood infiltration. The LIPO-PRO™ system is used to harvest your fat for mesenchymal stem cells. Harvest and Emcyte also have similar systems. Mesenchymal and hematopoietic stem cells accelerate healing faster than PRP alone.

Using your own tissues to heal represents a major health paradigm change and is the most exciting minimally invasive treatment currently available.

The goals of the stem cells from bone marrow and fat and PRP treatments are:

- Decrease pain to return to function and activity
- Minimal downtime
- No scars
- No complications, since you are using your own blood
- Resist injury reoccurrence
- Stabilized, resistant to further joint and tissue degeneration
- Accelerate healing process
- No pain medications
- No surgery

In addition to the Priapus Shot®, Cellular Medicine Association and Dr. Charles Runels have created not only the P Shot® but other incredible treatments for the face, breasts, hair, and female sexual dysfunction.

Vampire Facelift®:

- The physician uses a Hyaluronic Acid (HA) filler (like Restylane or Juvederm) in a very specific way to sculpt a younger appearing face, while still keeping the shape natural
- Then PRP is injected into the face
- Results in increased collagen and new blood flow creating a younger natural face.

In the first part of the Vampire Facelift® procedure, the doctor uses an HA filler (like Restylane® or Juvéderm®) in a particular way to sculpt a younger appearing face while still keeping the shape natural. Providers of the Vampire Facelift® procedure take into account the mathematics of beauty as defined by much research to avoid creating an unnatural shape. These ideas about the HA fillers are not commonly known even among the best of cosmetic surgeons and constitute part of the intellectual property protected by the trademarked name (Vampire Facelift®).After creating a younger and natural shape, the doctor harvests growth factors from the patient's blood (hence, the name Vampire). The growth factors are from the PRP, and they are what body would normally use to heal damaged tissue. The blood is drawn from the vein and put into a centrifuge and kit to separate whole blood into PRP.

Using numbing cream and a very small needle (for almost no pain), the PRP is put into the face in a particular way. These growth factors from PRP then activate stem cells already in the skin, tricking them into "thinking" there's been an injury, and new younger tissue is generated.

The effects of the procedure may improve for two to three months and last for at least one year.

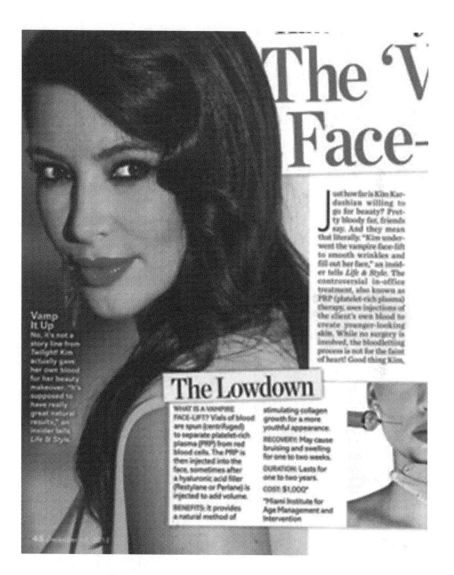

Vampire Facial®:

- A specific technique for micro-needling, followed by application of PRP
- Youthful, natural looking skin

What can you expect after three treatments, six weeks apart?

- Aging skin
  - ❖ Restores skin firmness and tightness to flaccid skin
  - ❖ Smooth away wrinkles, lines, folds, and crow's feet
  - ❖ Improves skin texture
  - ❖ Minimizes large pores
- Scars
  - ❖ Improves the appearance of scars from surgery, acne, chicken pox, keloids
- Pigmentation (brown spots)
  - ❖ Lightens pigmentation marks
- Cellulite and stretch marks
  - ❖ Improves the appearance of cellulite and stretch marks, new and old

The skin rejuvenation continues to improve for up to a year or more. The earlier and younger the treatment, the longer the improvements will last with more visible improvement.

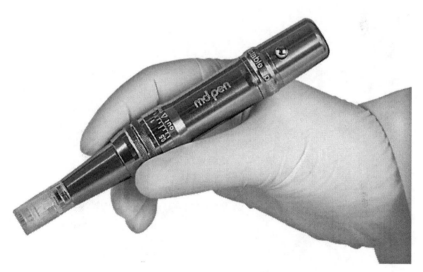

MDPen Microneedle

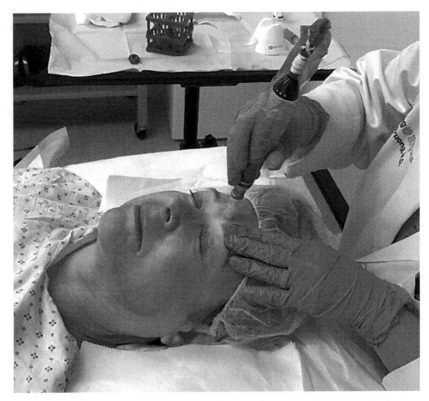

Vampire Facial®

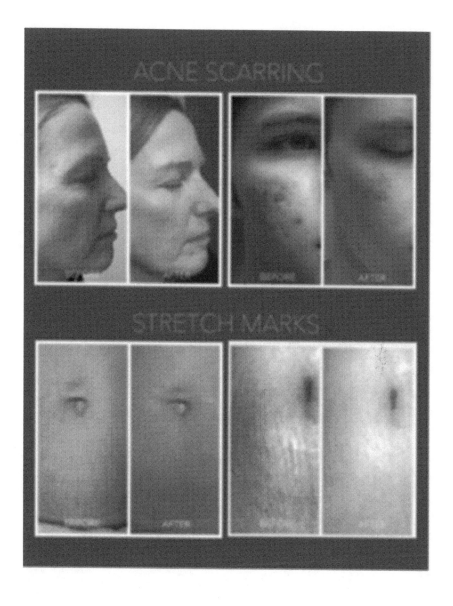

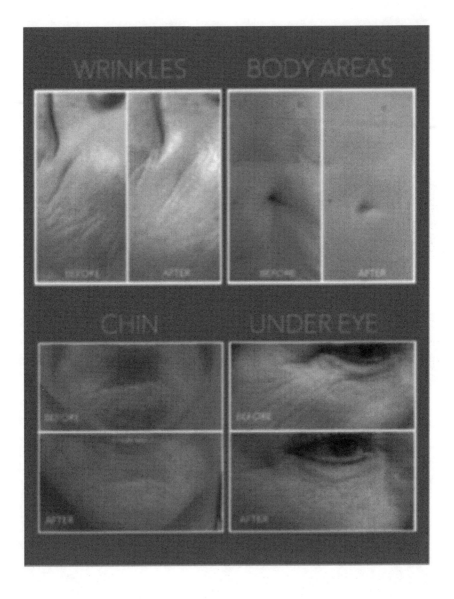

Vampire Breastlift®:

- Injection of PRP and Hyaluronic Acid filler into the cleavage of the breasts
- Improvements:
  - ❖ Skin color
  - ❖ The shape of the breast to be less collapsed and droopy
  - ❖ Sensation increased after breastfeeding, implants, other surgery, or aging
  - ❖ Corrected inverted nipple
  - ❖ Improves crinkling, crate-paper skin around the cleavage area

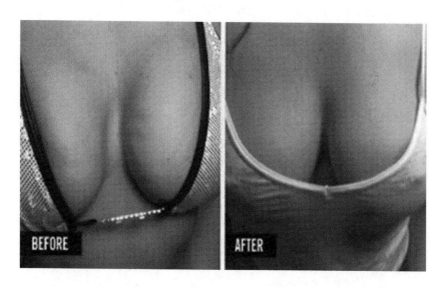

Vampire® Hair Regrowth:

- ❖ Platelet Rich Plasma (PRP) injected into the scalp to encourage new hair growth
- ❖ Effective for both male and female pattern hair loss
- ❖ Regrow hair in alopecia areata, eyebrow hypotrichosis and other patient cases with non-hereditary hair loss.

The Vampire® Hair Regrowth treatment takes about 90 minutes to complete. First, a blood sample is obtained which is specially processed to produce the PRP. A local anesthetic is then administered to numb the scalp treatment area completely. The PRP is then delivered via a series of injections over the full scalp or in a localized treatment area such as the eyebrows or beard.

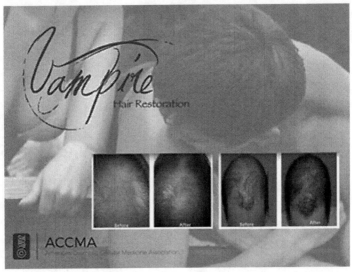

New hair growth can be seen as early as two months, but is typically evident between four to eight months and will continue to improve up to a year after treatment. Results have been maintained without additional injections for up two years in many patients, but no long-term data is yet available to conclude that this hair growth is permanent.

Orgasm Shot® or O Shot®:

The procedure is a very specific method of using blood-derived growth factors (PRP) to rejuvenate the vagina to help relieve women with urinary incontinence and sex problems. A specific protocol is followed, and if not done correctly results could be useless or worse. The names "Orgasm Shot" and "O-Shot" were awarded to Charles Runels, MD (the first to do the procedure) and are protected by US Patent & Trademark law.

Benefits:

- Injection of PRP into the vagina and clitoris
- Benefits:
  - ❖ Greater arousal from clitoral stimulation
  - ❖ Younger, smoother skin of the vulva (lips of the vagina).
  - ❖ A tighter introitus (vaginal opening)
  - ❖ Stronger orgasm
  - ❖ More frequent orgasm

- ❖ Increased sexual desire
- ❖ Increased ability to have a vaginal orgasm
- ❖ Decreased pain for those with dyspareunia (painful intercourse)
- ❖ Increased natural lubrication
- ❖ Decreased urinary incontinence

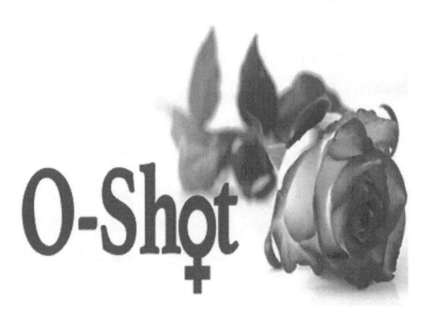

I am proud to be the provider of the Cellular Medicine Association. I have helped men and women with pain issues to facial, hair, breast restorations and sexual rejuvenation with PRP and mesenchymal regenerative cells.

Any physician or nurse practitioner who qualified, joined, and who continues in good standing with our group of O-Shot® and P Shot® providers will be listed on this website. Anyone who uses either name and who is not listed on this website is not a member of our group, is not certified to do the procedure, is violating trademark/patent laws, and should not be trusted.

To locate providers who are trained in these trademarked procedures, go to these websites:

- www.VampireFacelift.com
- www.OShot.com
- www.VampireFacial.com
- www.VampireBreastLift.com
- www.PriapusShot.com

REFERENCES

1. Original figure modified for this publication. Feldman HA, Goldstein I, Hatzichristou DG, et al. *Impotence and its medical and psychosocial correlates: results of the Massachusetts Male Aging Study.* J Urol 1994; 151:54.

2. Esposito K, Giugliano F, Di Palo C, et al. Effect of lifestyle changes on erectile dysfunction in obese men: a randomized controlled trial. JAMA 2004; 291:2978.

3. Table Hatzimouratidis K, Eardley I, Giuliano F, et al. European Association of Urology Guidelines on Male Sexual Dysfunction: *Erectile dysfunction and premature ejaculation.* 2015. Available at: uroweb.org/guideline/male-sexual-dysfunction/ (Accessed on April 16, 2015).

4. Krane RJ, Goldstein I, Saenz de Tejada I. *Impotence.* N Engl J Med 1989; 321:1648.

5. Karacan I, Williams RL, Thornby JI, Salis PJ. *Sleep-related penile tumescence as a function of age.* Am J Psychiatry 1975; 132:932.

6. Koskimäki J, Shiri R, Tammela T, et al. Regular intercourse protects against erectile dysfunction: Tampere Aging Male Urologic Study. Am J Med 2008; 121:592

7. Khera Mohit, Adaikan Ganesh, et al. Diagnosis and treatment of testosterone deficiency: *Recommendation from the fourth international consultation for sexual medicine* (ICSM 2015). J Sex Med 2016; 1787-1804

8. Calof OM, Singh AB, Lee ML, et al. Adverse events associated with testosterone replacement in middle age in older men: Met analysis of a randomized placebo controlled trials. J Gerontol A Biol Sci Med 2005; 60:1451-1457

9. Cunningham GR, Stephens-Shields AJ, Rosen RC, et al. *Testosterone Treatment and Sexual Function in Older Men With Low Testosterone Levels.* J Clin Endocrinol Metab 2016; 101:309

10. Lue TF. *Erectile dysfunction.* N Engl J Med 2000; 342:1802.

11. Montague DK, Angermeier KW. *Penile prosthesis implantation.* Urol Clin North Am 2001; 28:355

12. Lightfoot AJ, Rosevear HM, Kreder KJ. *Inflatable penile prostheses: an update.* Curr Opin Urol 2010; 20:459

13. Wilson, SK. *Penile prostheses at the millennium.* Contemporary Urology 2001; 13:35.

14. Quesada ET, Light JK. The AMS 700 inflatable penile prosthesis: long-term experience with the controlled expansion cylinders. J Urol 1993; 149:46.

15. Wilson SK, Delk JR 2nd. Inflatable penile implant infection: predisposing factors and treatment suggestions. J Urol 1995; 153:659.

16. Morgentaler A. *Male impotence.* Lancet 1999; 354:1713.

17. Jarow JP. Risk factors for penile prosthetic infection. J Urol 1996; 156:402.

18. Lewis, RW, McLaren, R. Reoperation for penile prosthesis implantation. Probl Urol 1993; 7:381. (DOI: 10.1159/000067984).

19. DePalma RG, Olding M, Yu GW, et al. *Vascular interventions for impotence: lessons learned.* J Vasc Surg 1995; 21:576.

20. Cookson MS, Phillips DL, Huff ME, Fitch WP 3rd. Analysis of microsurgical penile revascularization results by etiology of impotence. J Urol 1993; 149:1308.

21. Vardi Y, Gruenwald I, Gedalia U, et al. Evaluation of penile revascularization for erectile dysfunction: a 10-year follow-up. Int J Impot Res 2004; 16:181.

22. Kawanishi Y, Kimura K, Nakanishi R, et al. Penile revascularization surgery for arteriogenic erectile dysfunction: the long-term efficacy rate calculated bysurvival analysis. BJU Int 2004; 94:361.

23. Virag R. A New Treatment of Lapeyronie's Disease by Local Injections of Plasma Rich Platelets (PRP) and Hyaluronic Acid. Preliminary Results. e-mémoires de l'Académie Nationale de Chirurgie. 2014;13(3):96-100.

24. Safarinejad M. Safety and efficacy of coenzyme Q10 supplementation in early chronic Peyronie's disease: a double-blind, placebo-controlled randomized study. International Journal of Impotence Research. 2010;22(5):298-309.

25. Paulis G. Efficacy of vitamin E in the conservative treatment of Peyronie's disease: legend or reality? A controlled study of 70 cases. Andrology. 2013;1(1):120-128.

26. Raheem A. The role of vacuum pump therapy to mechanically straighten the penis in Peyronie's disease. BJU Int. 2016; 117(4):E7.

27. Levine L. Peyronie's disease: contemporary review of non-surgical treatment. Transl. Androl. Urol. 2013;2(1):39-44.

28. Pahlajani G,Raina R, Jones S, Ali M, and Zippe C. Vacuum erection devices revisited: Its emerging role in the treatment of erectile dysfunction and early penile rehabilitation following prostate cancer therapy. J Sex Med 2012; 9:1182–1189.

29. Lue T. The Challenges of Peyronie's disease. Translational Andrology & Urology. 2012;1(S1):PS 9.

30. Kalyvianakis D, Hatzichristou D. Low-Intensity Shockwave Therapy Improves Hemodynamic Parameters in Patients With Vasculogenic Erectile Dysfunction: A Triplex Ultrasonography-Based Sham-Controlled Trial. J Sex Med 2017; 14: 891-897.

31. Thompson WR, Scott A, Loghmani MT, et al. Understanding mechanobiology: physical therapists as a force in mechanotherapy and musculoskeletal regenerative rehabilitation. Phys Ther 2015:96(4):560-9.

32. Daar AS, Greenwood HL. *A proposed definition of regenerative medicine.* J Tissue Eng Regen Med 2007:1(3):179-84.

33. Huang C, Holfeld J, Schaden W, et al. Mechanotherapy: revisiting physical therapy and recruiting mechanobiology for a new era in medicine. Trends Mol Med 2013:19(9):555-64.

34. Chiquet M, Renedo AS, Huber F, et al. How do fibroblasts translate mechanical signals into changes in extracellular matrix productions? Matrix Biol 2003:22(1):73-80.

35. Feldman HA, Goldstein I, Hatzichristou DG, et al: Impotence and its medical and psychosocial correlates: Results of the Massachusetts Male Aging Study. J Urol, 1994;151:54–61.

36. Johannes CB, Araujo AB, Feldman HA, et al: Incidence of erectile dysfunction in men 40 to 69 years old: Longitudinal results from the Massachusetts Male Aging Study. J Urol, 2000;163:460–463.

37. Laumann EO, Paik A, Rosen RC: Sexual dysfunction in the United States: Prevalence and predictors. JAMA, 1999;281:537–544.

38. Kalyvianakis D, Hatzichristou D. Low-IntensityShockwave Therapy Improves Hemodynamic Parameters in Patients With Vasculogenic ErectileDysfunction: A Triplex Ultrasonography-Based Sham-Controlled Trial. J Sex Med 2017;14:891-897.

39. C.S. Kumar, *Combined Treatment of Injecting Platelet Rich Plasma With Vacuum Pump for Penile Enlargement*, , Journal of Sexual Medicine January 2017, Volume 14, Issue 1, Supplement 1, Page S78.

40. J Urol. 2003 Aug;170(2 Pt 2):S24-9; discussion S29-30.*Vasculogenic erectile dysfunction: newer therapeutic strategies.* Siroky MB, Azadzoi KM.

41. Casabona, F., Gambelli, I., Casabona, F. et al. Int Urol Nephrol (2017) 49: 573. Autologous platelet-rich plasma (PRP) in chronic penile lichen sclerosus: the impact on tissue repair and patient quality of life. https://doi.org/10.1007/s11255-017-1523-0.

42. Shamloul R, Ghanem H. *Erectile dysfunction.* Lancet 2013; 381:153.

43. Grant P, Jackson G, Baig I, Quin J. *Erectile dysfunction in general medicine.* Clin Med 2013; 13:136.

44. Bacon CG, Mittleman MA, Kawachi I, et al. Sexual function in men older than 50 years of age: results from the health professionals follow-up study. Ann Intern Med 2003; 139:161.

45. Siroky M. Vasculogenic erectile dysfunction: newer therapeutic strategies. J Urol. 2003;170(2 Pt 2):S24-9.

46. Garcia MM, Fandel TM, Lin G, Shindel AW, Banie L, LinC-S, and Lue TF. Treatment of erectile dysfunction in the obese type 2 diabetic ZDF rat with adipose tissue-derived stem cells. J Sex Med 2010;7:89–98.

47. Rogers R. Intracavernosal vascular endothelial growth factor (VEGF) injection and adeno-associated virus-mediated VEGF gene therapy prevent and reverse venogenic erectile dysfunction in rats. International Journal of Impotence Research. 2003;15:S24-9.

48. Lamina S, Agbanusi E, Nwacha RC. Effects of Aerobic Exercise in the Management of Erectile Dysfunction: A Meta Analysis Study on Randomized Controlled Trials. Ethiopian Journal of Health Sciences. 2011;21(3):195-201.

49. Nikolai S. Erection rehabilitation following prostatectomy--current strategies and future directions. Nature Reviews Urology. 2016;13(.):216-225.

50. Sellers T, Dineen M, Wilson SK. Vacuum protocol and cylinders that lengthen allow implantation of longer, inflatable prosthesis. Toronto, ON: (Abst) Society of Sexual Medicine; 2008.

51. Raynor M. Dorsal Penile Nerve Block Prior to Inflatable Penile Prosthesis Placement: A Randomized, Placebo-Controlled Trial. The Journal of Sexual Medicine. 2012;9(11):2975-2979.

52. Sanchez-Gonzales J. *Platelet-Rich Plasma Peptides: Key for Regeneration.* International Journal of Peptides. 2012;10:1-10.

53. Taylor D. A systematic review of the use of platelet-rich plasma in sports medicine as a new treatment for tendon and ligament injuries. Clin J Sport Med. 2011; 21(4):344-52.

54. Yuan T, Zhang C-Q, Wang JH-C. *Augmenting tendon and ligament repair with platelet-rich plasma (PRP).* Muscles, Ligaments and Tendons Journal. 2013;3(3):139-149.

55. Sell S. A case report on the use of sustained release platelet-rich plasma for the treatment of chronic pressure ulcers. The Journal of Spinal Cord Medicine. 2011;34(1):122-7.

56. Conde-Montero, E., Horcajada-Reales, C., Clavo, P., Delgado-Sillero, I. and Suárez-Fernández, R. (2014), *Neuropathic ulcers in leprosy treated with intralesional platelet-rich plasma.* Int Wound J. doi:10.1111/iwj.12359.

57. Ding X. The effect of platelet-rich plasma on cavernous nerve regeneration in a rat model. Asian J Androl. 2009;11(2):215-21.

58. Ding X. *Platelet-rich plasma on the Cavernous Nerve Regeneration.* Chinese Medical journal. 2008;88(36):2578-2580.

59. Rene' Y. Safety of Intracavernous Bone Marrow-Mononuclear Cells for Postradical Prostatectomy Erectile Dysfunction: An Open Dose-Escalation Pilot Study. European Urology. 2016;69(6):988-991.

60. Fandel T. Recruitment of Intracavernously Injected Adipose-Derived Stem Cells to the Major Pelvic Ganglion Improves Erectile Function in a Rat Model of Cavernous Nerve Injury. European Urology. 2012;61(1):201-210.

61. Singh S. Role of platelet-rich plasma in chronic alopecia areata: Our centre experience. Indian Journal of Plastic Surgery. 2015;48(1):57-9.

62. Goldstein A. ISSVD 2015 Abstracts. Autologous Platelet Rich Plasma (PRP) Intradermal Injections for the Treatment of Vulvar Lichen Sclerosus. Journal of Lower Genital Tract Disease. 2015; 19(3):S1-S25.

63. Goldstein A., Runels C. Intradermal Injection of autologous platelet-rich plasma for the treatment of vulvar Lichen sclerosus. Journal of the American Academy of Dermatology. 2017; 76(1):158-160.

64. Zaman H. Association of psychological factors, patients' knowledge, and management among patients with erectile dysfunction. Patient Preference and Adherence. 2016;10:807.

65. Kupelian V, Page ST, Araujo AB, et al. Low sex hormone-binding globulin, total testosterone, and symptomatic androgen deficiency are associated with development of the metabolic syndrome in nonobese men. J Clin Endocrinol Metab 2006; 91:843.

66. Laaksonen DE, Niskanen L, Punnonen K, et al. Testosterone and sex hormone-binding globulin predict the metabolic syndrome and diabetes in middle-aged men. Diabetes Care 2004; 27:1036.

67. Oh JY, Barrett-Connor E, Wedick NM, et al. Endogenous sex hormones and the development of type 2 diabetes in older men and women: the Rancho Bernardo study. Diabetes Care 2002; 25:55.

68. Kaplan SA, Johnson-Levonas AO, Lin J, et al. Elevated high sensitivity C-reactive protein levels in aging men with low testosterone. Aging Male 2010; 13:108.

69. Selvin E1, Burnett AL, Platz EA. Prevalence and risk factors for erectile dysfunction in the US. Am J Med. 2007 Feb;120(2):151-7.

70. Wu FC, Tajar A, Pye SR, et al. Hypothalamic-pituitary-testicular axis disruptions in older men are differentially linked to age and modifiable risk factors: the European Male Aging Study. J Clin Endocrinol Metab 2008; 93:2737.

71. Bremner WJ, Vitiello MV, Prinz PN. Loss of circadian rhythmicity in blood testosterone levels with aging in normal men. J Clin Endocrinol Metab 1983; 56:1278.

Dr. Anne Truong, author of *Erectile Dysfunction Fix*, has helped thousands of men to ease erectile dysfunction (ED) and enjoy intimate relationships once more. Her treatments involve Platelets Rich Plasma (PRP), which uses the body's own blood and innate healing abilities to mend injuries and treat ED. Personally taught by Dr. Charles Runels, the inventor of the Priapus Shot® used to administer PRP, she has found this method to be a natural alternative to widespread ED remedies, without the lasting side effects of many existing medications. In addition to treating patients for erectile dysfunction, joint pain, and spine discomfort, Dr. Truong also teaches other doctors to effectively use the PRP technique.

Dr. Anne Truong is Board Certified in Physical Medicine and Rehabilitation, along with Electrodiagnostic Medicine. Dr. Truong earned her bachelor's from the University of California, Berkley and her medical doctorate from the University of Nevada, School of Medicine. Dr. Truong continued her training in Internal Medicine at The University of California, Irvine, and completed her residency in Physical Medicine and Rehabilitation at Baylor College of Medicine in Houston, Texas. Dr. Truong then continued on as an assistant professor at Baylor College of Medicine in Houston, Texas, teaching Physical Medicine and Rehabilitation to physicians in training.

After a few years, Dr. Truong relocated to Fredericksburg, Virginia, to start her medical practice in areas of pain management and rehabilitation, functional medicine, regenerative medicine, and cosmetic and sexual medicine. Dr. Truong is the sole founder and owner of Truong Rehabilitation Center, where she serves as president. She has over twenty years of medical expertise and has taught physicians globally on regenerative, cosmetic and sexual medicine. Dr. Truong currently serves as the Ambassador for Women Entrepreneurs Day Organization at United Nations and was awarded 2018 Entrepreneur of the Year from the Chamber of Commerce. Dr. Truong resides with her husband and two children in the Fredericksburg area.

Visit her online at www.truongrehab.com.

Made in the USA
Middletown, DE
28 February 2024